Distribution, publication, and copying in any form are prohibited and subject to damages.

TEN HYPNOSES

Copying, publishing, and sharing with third parties are only permitted with the written consent of the author. Please observe the notes on copyright and usage.

Distribution, publication, and copying in any form are prohibited and subject to damages.

Copying, publishing, and sharing with third parties are only permitted with the written consent of the author. Please observe the notes on copyright and usage.

Distribution, publication, and copying in any form are prohibited and subject to damages.

Ingo Michael Simon

TEN HYPNOSES

5

COPING WITH THE PAST

Copying, publishing, and sharing with third parties are only permitted with the written consent of the author. Please observe the notes on copyright and usage.

Distribution, publication, and copying in any form are prohibited and subject to damages.

© 2024 Ingo Michael Simon
All rights reserved.
Independently published
www.ingosimon.com

Important Notes for Urgent Attention:
The contents of this book are based on the practical experiences of the author with hypnosis applications and psychotherapy in a trance state. Although the author has strived for the utmost care, errors or misunderstandings in the presentation cannot be completely excluded. Therapeutic work with people and the application of hypnosis are solely the responsibility of the hypnotist. It cannot be ruled out that parts of this book may be misunderstood or that the application of a presented procedure may cause an undesirable reaction in the client. The author also assumes no co-responsibility if work with a client is carried out with reference to the statements in this book.

The Author:
Ingo Michael Simon studied psychology and education and is a hypnotherapist with practices in southwestern Germany and Switzerland. With the help of hypnosis-supported psychotherapy, he primarily treats people with persistent psychological conditions. His practice focuses on anxiety disorders, pathological compulsions, and psychosomatic illnesses. His therapeutic offerings mainly include classical and modern hypnosis applications and the dreamland therapy he developed himself.

Copying, publishing, and sharing with third parties are only permitted with the written consent of the author. Please observe the notes on copyright and usage.

Notes on Copyright and Usage

Copying, publishing, and sharing with third parties is prohibited and only permitted with the written consent of the author. Please observe the following copyright and usage guidelines.

This work has been carefully crafted and created to the best of the author's knowledge and personal experience. It comprises text templates and application guidelines for professional hypnosis sessions. The author is a licensed psychotherapist with extensive experience in psychotherapy, coaching, and personal training using hypnotic techniques and methods. Nevertheless, the author and the publisher assume no liability for the accuracy of information, instructions, and advice, nor for any typographical errors. The author and publisher accept no responsibility or liability for the application of these texts and recommendations with clients or patients, nor for any potential consequences or unexpected reactions. It is expressly noted that the application of therapeutic and advisory techniques and formulations lies solely and entirely within the responsibility of the practitioner. This also applies to adherence to the boundaries of legally regulated medical and therapeutic practices. The fact that a book containing action proposals is freely available for sale does not imply that its application with clients or patients is permitted for everyone.

Distribution, publication, and copying in any form are prohibited and subject to damages.

Copying, publishing, and sharing with third parties are only permitted with the written consent of the author. Please observe the notes on copyright and usage.

Distribution, publication, and copying in any form are prohibited and subject to damages.

Table of contents

Introduction 9

#1 11

#2 16

#3 21

#4 26

#5 31

#6 36

#7 40

#8 45

#9 50

#10 55

Overview of All Titles in the Series "Ten Hypnoses" 60

Copying, publishing, and sharing with third parties are only permitted with the written consent of the author. Please observe the notes on copyright and usage.

Distribution, publication, and copying in any form are prohibited and subject to damages.

Copying, publishing, and sharing with third parties are only permitted with the written consent of the author. Please observe the notes on copyright and usage.

Introduction

The series "Ten Hypnoses" is very well known in Germany, Austria, and Switzerland as a collection of texts for therapeutic work and is used by numerous psychotherapeutic practices, doctors, therapists, coaches, and other helping professionals. I am pleased to now be able to offer these texts in other countries as well.

Most therapists have their own methods for inducing and deepening trance as well as for exiting trance. Therefore, I have focused on the main part of the hypnosis. The texts in this book can be integrated as the main part into any hypnosis process.

The texts in this collection use various hypnosis techniques. I will not explain these in detail, as I assume that users have the appropriate training. It is also not necessary to understand the exact structure or functioning of the different parts. The texts can simply be read aloud, and they will have their effect.

Decide for yourself which text best suits your client or patient at any given time. You can also combine passages from different texts. It is not about using all ten hypnoses in sequence. It is a selection of possibilities.

I want to emphasize that books cannot replace therapy. Psychotherapy or other therapeutic treatments involve much more. A careful diagnosis is the necessary basis for deciding on the use of methods, including whether hypnosis or one of my texts should be used. Even in this case, preparatory discussions, follow-up discussions during the session, and of course, a therapeutic concept for the sequence of sessions and the content approaches are essential parts of therapy. This cannot and should not be achieved with a collection of texts.

In any case, I wish you much success in your work and I am pleased if my text templates can contribute in a small way.

Ingo Michael Simon

#1

You have confronted your past and you know what happened... ... Now you are ready to let go of the past... ... To send it where it belongs... ... to a time that has passed and no longer plays a role today... ... Your decision is correct, because you have already learned everything from your past that you could learn... ... Everything is done and completed... ... So you can always remember if you want to, but you no longer need the past... ... It is over... ... Earlier you thought it would not be easy to let go of the past... ... Today you know exactly that you can let go of what you have understood... ... And you have understood the past enough... ...

So let's go... ... I will accompany you now as you let go... ... Imagine that the past is only a memory in your thoughts... ... nothing more, as it is already over... ... What you held onto were your feelings about past events... ... but you no longer need those... ... Today you let go... ...

Imagine that you can simply let go of all your thoughts with your breathing... ... as if you could just exhale your thoughts… … And you can do just that… … It is truly amazing that this is possible… … We do it every day… … With a long breath, we let go of tension, anger, frustrations many times a day… … We simply exhale and let go… … just like you are doing now… … With each breath, you let something go… …

When you inhale, you feel the air in your nose… … you can feel the airflow up to your eyes… … While doing this, imagine your breath flowing through your entire head, touching all your thoughts… … And your breath simply carries away all disturbing thoughts of the past and exhales them… … like an inner cleansing… …

So you exhale and let go of past events… … all the situations and scenes that once impressed you so much and occupied you for so long… … You exhale slowly and long to really let go now… … You exhale and let go of the old events… … You have learned everything you need… … You exhale and let go… … You exhale slowly and long to really let go now… …

You exhale and let go of people from your past… … even if they still play a role in your life today… … Today is today and yesterday was sometime ago... ... You exhale slowly and long to really let go now... ... You let go of the past of these people now... ... You exhale and let go of these people now... ... and with them all the sorrow and pain you had in contact or dealings with them... ... You exhale slowly and long to really let go now... ...

You exhale and let go of old thought patterns that you no longer need today... ... You have long understood what is important today and which values matter to you today... ... You exhale slowly and long to really let go now... ... Many things you thought before are no longer suitable today... ... Today is today and today you simply let go of old thought patterns... ... This creates space for new creativity... ... for new thinking and new actions... ... You exhale slowly and long to really let go now... ...

You exhale and let go of old feelings... ... You make it clear to yourself which feelings play a role in your present... ... which feelings actually relate to the present... ... You exhale slowly and long to really let go now... ... Today you let go of old feelings... ... right at this moment... ... You exhale and let go of old feelings... ... You exhale slowly and long to really let go now... ...

Now you have found space for new paths... ... Now you focus on your present and the challenges it brings... ... You exhale and feel a deep strength within you... ... You feel a very deep strength within you... ...

... ... Now feel your breathing very consciously and follow the rhythm of your breath... ... With each breath, you can let go more and find new freedom... ... Freedom that you can fill with your new impulses... ... again and again you let go... ... with each breath... ... You let go of past events and feel the new freedom within you... ... You let go of past people and feel the new freedom within you... ... You let go of past thought patterns and feel the new freedom within you... ... You let go of past feelings and feel the new freedom within you... ...

All these words are deeply anchored in your subconscious... ... Everything is imprinted deeply in your feeling... ... So every day, if you want, you can breathe specifically for your letting go and breathe for your inner freedom... ... Whenever you consciously and deliberately exhale slowly and long, because you want to let go, you immediately feel the inner liberation... ... the lightness... ...

You simply breathe slowly and long and feel your letting go... ...

Whenever you feel that old thoughts might come back, you simply breathe slowly and long... ... slowly and long... ... and let go while doing so... ... just like today... ... exactly like today... ...

#2

Today is the day of change... ... For far too long you have held on to the past... ... you have struggled with fate... ... you have often felt guilty because you blamed yourself for much of what happened in the past... ... So often you have thought about everything... ... so often wondered how it could be today and how you could feel if everything had gone differently... ...

... ... Then there was always the bitter realization that the past cannot be changed... ... no matter how long you think about it... ... no matter how many reproaches you make to yourself or others... ... no matter how much you wish for it... ... what is past is past... ... and the past is over... ... But thinking about it makes sense because you can learn from the past... ... you might do things differently in the future, react earlier... ... find other ways... ... maybe even take flight in time... ... You can learn from the past... ... and that is exactly what you have already done... ... You have confronted the events and occurrences again and again... ...

perhaps you have repeatedly tried to better understand everything or to learn your lesson from the experiences... ...

... ... But if you think about it now, you quickly realize that this learning process is already completed... ... You have learned everything you could learn... ... maybe you do not understand many things, cannot comprehend or accept the actions of other people... ... but you have learned and understood enough... ... Now it is time to move into the present... ... to arrive in the moment of the present, because only then can you experience and shape the present... ...

... ... It is an inner step that you are taking now... ... maybe even a leap... ... a leap into the present, because here you are needed... ... here you can apply what you have learned... ... here you can shape and influence... ... here you can ensure that things will be different from now on... ... Now you can take control of your life again and actively shape it... ... free from old patterns... ... free from old feelings... ... Here and today it is up to you... ... Here and today your actions count... ... Live in the moment now... ... Live in the moment now... ...

… … You firmly resolve to perceive the moment… … to feel how you are doing now… … right at this moment… … You look within yourself… … and if the thought arises that you are suffering now because you are thinking about the past, you immediately realize that this is not the feeling of the moment but a feeling of the past… … So, how are you now? … … Consider an answer that you can give yourself in thought… … How are you now, in exactly this moment… … in your present? … …

… … You prepare yourself that it is all about this question… … about the question of how you are in the moment of the present… … exactly in this moment… … only that matters… …

… … Maybe you think that is too little… … You are right… … We all have to act because life goes on… … we have to plan because we have to shape the future… … which will soon be the present… …

… … The second of the present, exactly this one moment you are in now, will be the past in the next second, over… … You can only experience the present… … But the future is in the next second already your new present… … You are moving towards the future that will become the present... ... to the moment that counts... ... But the past will never come back... ... It is over... ... It is over... ... You live in the moment of the present... ... You act now and thereby also shape the future... ... All your abilities... ... all your strength and creativity are at your disposal... ... Live in the moment and look within yourself... ... Feel what you are feeling now... ... Feel what your body is feeling now... ... Think what your thoughts are thinking now... ... Decide what is important now... ... Become free to feel exactly what is there now... ...

Enjoy the moment... ... enjoy the moment... ... Isn't it wonderful how free you feel when you really focus entirely on the moment, just like now... ... Truly amazing how well you succeed in focusing only on the present now... ... only on yourself in this one moment... ... only on yourself in this one moment... ... So let this feeling become clearer... ... Become more and more aware in your feeling, being entirely in the present... ... free from old chains and patterns... ... free from old thoughts... ... You can increasingly feel how liberating it is to be completely in the moment... ... now in this moment very intensely, and if you want, again and again... ... Feel more and more clearly how liberating and light you feel... ... how open you become to your

own feeling... ... entirely in the moment of the present... ... entirely with yourself... ... entirely with yourself... ... just like that... ... exactly like that... ...

You think of a ritual that you can use every day to come back to this beautiful state... ... perhaps through a short meditation... ... or a breathing exercise, where you breathe calmly with your eyes closed... ... and imagine taking a big inner step into the present... ... And whenever you close your eyes and imagine taking a big step, you immediately come into this state of freedom that you feel now... ... Your deep inner self knows that your ritual of closing your eyes and imagining taking a big step is meant to bring you from the past immediately into the moment of the present... ... with a short meditation or a short breathing exercise... ... simply by closing your eyes and wishing to come into the present with all your mindfulness... ... You find your ritual that will bring you back to the present again and again... ... just like now... ... exactly like now... ...

#3

The following version of a hypnosis main part works with an anchor in the form of a handy note with the word "Let Go" printed on it. An anchor is a trigger that is supposed to create a certain feeling or awaken a certain thought. We want to help the client use a "reminder card" to quickly adjust to letting go when they notice in everyday life that the past is influencing their actions. We discuss this with the client before the session and prepare the reminder card. It can be a labeled business card or something similar. The card is prepared and given to the client to hold lightly in their hand or place on their body, for example, on the solar plexus. They should carry the card with them after the hypnosis, in their pants pocket or jacket pocket.

You have the goal of finally consigning the past to the past... ... to send it to the place of memory and leave it there... ... because that's where the past belongs... ... You can recall the events and experiences in your memory, but they should not come into the present... ... because the present belongs only to you... ... It was your own holding on that led to the past determining your present so strongly, but that had to be... ... It is important that we hold on just as long as we need to process and understand the experienced... ... You have now reached this point... ... You have processed and you have understood... ... Therefore, now is the right time to let go... ... to let go of the past and send it to the place of a memory... ...

... ... You have decided that you want to let go... ... You have understood that it is you who must turn your intentions into truth... ... You know that it is you who makes your success... ... and you are ready for it... ... You are ready to give everything necessary to become inwardly free... ... free from old burdens of the past... ... You have the potential for this... ... you have the strength you need for this... ...

But you want more... ... You want to be able to access your qualities and abilities at any time and in full... ... You want to be able to let go again and again... ... especially when you might hold on to the past too much again... ... and suddenly notice it... ...

You know the important word, the decisive one... ... Let go... ... It is like a message to yourself... ... Let go... ... It is like a reminder... ... Let go... ... like a prompt that only you can give yourself... ... Let go... ... Let go... ...

You have this card with exactly this inscription, the card shows your task... ... Let go... ... You feel this inner strength growing within you... ... You know that you can accomplish anything... ... your will and readiness grow with every breath and become clearer with every breath... ... Let go... ... The card shows it to you every day... ... It shows you your task, which you can always carry with you... ... Let go... ... It helps you become stronger every day and finally be free again and again... ... As soon as even the slightest doubt arises within you, you immediately take the card in your hand and read the inscription clearly, you look at it... ... Let go... ... Then you immediately feel the effect, you feel that this is your truth... ... You do it every day... ... ... You simply let go of the past... ... You simply let go of the past... ...

The card shows it to you every day... It shows you your own attitude, which you can always carry with you... ... It helps you through difficult moments... ... As soon as even the slightest doubt arises within you, you immediately take the card in your hand and look at it... ... Let go... ... Then you immediately feel the effect, you feel that this is your truth... ...

... ... Now take your reminder card consciously in your hand... ... Hold it firmly... ... Did you notice that you are holding on to something again? ... ... This time you are holding on to letting go... ... and as incredible and paradoxical as it may sound... ... That is a good holding on... ... holding on to your goal of letting go... ... holding on to the fact that you are important to yourself... ... holding on to your goal of freeing yourself... ... holding on to the fact that there is nothing more important to you than finally letting go of the past... ... holding on only to the moment of the present... ... holding on only to the moment of the present... ... In the next second, the present is over... ... and everything that is over, you let go... ... The card you feel between your fingers reminds you of this... ... it helps you let go... ... it helps you to be free and to take new paths... ... free and open to the future... ... free and open... ... every day... ...

... ... [Ask the client now to open the eyes and read the word in trance. This enhances the effect. Opening the eyes

is a fractionation that can be done without special announcement or counting. Every person can open their eyes in trance. In a stable and deep trance, it is somewhat difficult because the client is tired and sluggish. Just stay suggestive until the eyes are opened and the card is read.]
... ...

... ... Consciously feel the reminder card between your fingers and if you want, open your eyes briefly and look at the card... ... open your eyes and read what is written there... ... Let go... ...

... ... Now close your eyes again and let the read word work deep within you... ... very deep... ...

You still feel the card between your fingers... ... You know that it can remind you every day to become free by letting go... ... Whenever you take the card in your hand and read it, you immediately feel that you become inwardly calmer and freer... ... calmer and freer... ... Whenever you carry the card with you, you feel inwardly calmer and freer... ... calmer and freer... ... It happens by itself because your inner self knows that this card reminds you of what you did today... ... your own liberation... ...

#4

The following hypnosis session works with a physical anchor. An anchor is a trigger that is supposed to create a certain feeling or awaken a certain thought. We want to help the client produce the feeling of freedom from the past with a light pressure on the left hand (on the pad below the thumb). We discuss this with the client before the session and show them the spot they should press on. During the hypnosis session, we then set the anchor. It is important to connect the pressing of the thumb pad in a state of calm with the already existing feeling of inner freedom. The client must absolutely feel light and free during this session. This must be absolutely certain, otherwise it will not work. In case of doubt, ask if they feel the inner freedom. If not, deepen the relaxation and encourage the feeling of freedom with suggestions before setting the anchor.

You finally want to be free... ... This goal is your goal, and you have already done a lot for it... ... Today you can take another, very big and very decisive step... ... Today you can set your deep inner self to feel truly free... ... free from old connections to long-gone events... ... free from old anger... ... free from old disappointments... ... free from the desire for reparation... ... free from the desire to change or undo everything... ... You can also set your body to end the holding on to the past now... ... Both are directly connected... ... As soon as your inner self is ready to let go, your body signals you relaxation because it lets go too... ... To let go again and again, you can bring your body into a calm state and thus inform your inner self that it can let go now... ...

.. ... We are working with an anchor today, as we have already discussed... ... You already carry this anchor on your body... ... your left hand is the anchor triggered by your right hand... ... But we will get to that a little later... ... To use the anchor one hundred percent, find the best position now to trigger it... ... Reach with your right hand to your left and feel the pad with your fingers... ... very lightly... ... very gently... ... Decide whether you want to grasp with your thumb and index finger or with your thumb and middle finger... ... maybe you have another way... ... Do it in the way you can best grasp your thumb pad... ... [Wait until the client finds a good grip; ask again if they don't "join in" right away]... ... Wonderful... ... This works best... ... very good... ... And now let go of your hand again and place both hands loosely beside your body... ...

... ... Now it is time to find a very deep inner peace... ... deeper than ever before... ... You go deeper and deeper into this state of inner peace... ... as if

you could sink into yourself... ... You let go of all thoughts... ... You let go of the memory of the past... ... You let go of the anger of the past... ... You let go of the disappointment... ... You let go of the desire for reparation... ... and you pay very close attention to your body feeling... ... You feel how calm you are at this moment... ... You are really calm and feel free now in this moment... ... truly free... ... Isn't it remarkable how easily you can feel this feeling so clearly? ... ... As soon as you have made a decision, you can act... ... At this moment, you make it perfectly clear to yourself that you have already made a decision... ... You have decided to be free and look forward... ... to shape the present and move towards the future... ... to take good care of yourself... ... So you don't need more than a single second to act on your decision... ...

From now on, you simply do what is necessary to make your decision a reality... ... to feel that you are actually free whenever you want... ... just like now... ... Right now, in this very moment, you can feel that you are free... ...

You feel the deep desire within you to feel this feeling again and again whenever you are disturbed or limited by memories... ...

... ... You have decided, so you can act... ... In the word 'act' is the word 'hand'... ... Now you can actually act... ... Reach for your left hand as soon as you truly feel free inside... ...

... ... [Wait. Give the client time. Encourage again after 30 seconds if needed, or ask if they feel free. If not, deepen the relaxation and promote the feeling of freedom with suggestions before setting the anchor.] ...

... ... Do it now as you have practiced... ... Grasp your left hand and focus on your inner feeling of freedom... ... If you think the feeling of freedom should become even clearer, just let it become even clearer and more intense in your feeling... ... even more intense... ... with even more mindfulness and care for yourself... ... just like that... ... just like that... ... You can do it... ...

... ... And now let this feeling become very conscious... ... and press the pad of your left hand... ... and again... ... press... ... Your inner self sets itself so that exactly this pressing of the thumb pad is the signal to immediately feel that you are actually free... ... Whenever you press your thumb pad, you feel free and feel the need to take care of yourself... ... to take yourself seriously... ... to be important to yourself... ... Your body is relaxed and also your hands are completely calm... ... Your body has understood how your anchor works... ... It has already stored it for you so that you can use it again and again... ...

... ... Whenever you press your thumb pad, you are really free and feel the need to be only in the present and to shape it... ... to take yourself seriously... ... to be important to yourself... ... Soon it will become natural for you to press your thumb pad or massage it, it works just like that... ... exactly like now... ... You have decided... ... You have acted...

#5

You know the difficulties you have had until today. You also know your goals... ... You know what you want to achieve... ... You want to end holding on to the past... ... want to break the chains of old patterns and entanglements... ... want to feel strength and hope again... ... You want to live again... ...

... ... For this, it is necessary to change your thoughts and feelings... ... If you think about it, you understand that your bitterness and anger were mainly the result of disturbing thoughts and feelings... ... So you want to let go of these disturbing thoughts and feelings... ... Maybe you are already curious about how that works... ... Imagine that every single thought is a small colored pearl that is in your head... ... All feelings are also small pearls in your head... ... So you only need to find and let go of the disturbing thoughts and feelings... ... You recognize them by their color... ... Your breathing helps you with this... ...

... ... Let's consider, for example, your disappointment with the experiences and events of the past... ... your unfulfilled wishes... ... your sadness... ... So you can imagine that all thoughts and all feelings that belong to your disappointment are blue... ... In your head, there are therefore many small blue pearls that you can let go of... ... You do this through your breathing... ... You inhale and the air flows through your head... ... You see it before your inner eye... ... The air collects all the blue thoughts and feelings and carries them with it... ... And you exhale them... ... Like soap bubbles, they come out of your nose and float through the room... ... lots of blue soap bubbles... ... and one after the other, they burst... ... And you continue... ... You inhale and collect all the blue thoughts and feelings... ... As soap bubbles, you exhale them... ... They float through the room and dissolve... ... You repeat this with every breath. Your disappointment dissolves more and more... ...

... ... Your deep inner self is already letting new thoughts arise... ... You feel hope in the process... ... This happens by itself. You simply continue to breathe and observe the blue soap bubbles dissolving... ... and hope arises... ...

... ... Next, let's consider your bitterness, your anger... ... You know what it's like... ... You have often had thoughts of revenge or reparation... ... have struggled with fate and felt the injustice you experienced as a punishment... ... All thoughts and feelings that deal with bitterness or anger or lead to bitterness and anger are red... ... In your head, there are therefore many red pearls that you can let go of... ... You inhale and collect all the red thoughts and feelings... ... And you exhale them... ... Like soap bubbles, they come out of your nose and float through the room... ... lots of red soap bubbles... ... and one after the other, they burst... ... And you continue... ... You inhale and collect all the red thoughts and feelings... ... As soap bubbles, you exhale them... ... They float through the room and dissolve... ... You repeat this with every breath... ...

... ... Your deep inner self is already letting new thoughts arise. In place of anger, gentleness and calm arise... ... This happens by itself... ... You simply continue to breathe and observe the red soap bubbles dissolving... ... Gentleness and calm become stronger... ... Gentleness and calm become stronger... ...

... ... Now consider your feelings of guilt... ... because you have often accused yourself... ... maybe you even think now that you did something wrong or loaded guilt on yourself... ... All thoughts and feelings associated with guilt have the color yellow... ... In your head, there are therefore many yellow pearls that you can let go of... ... You inhale and collect all the yellow thoughts and feelings... ... And you exhale them... ... Like soap bubbles, they come out of your nose and float through the room... ... lots of yellow soap bubbles... ... and one after the other, they burst... ... And you continue... ... You inhale and collect all the yellow thoughts and feelings... ... As soap bubbles, you exhale them... ... They float through the room and dissolve... ... You repeat this with every breath... ...

... ... Your deep inner self is already letting new thoughts arise. You become free and recognize that you are innocent... ... This happens by itself... ... You simply continue to breathe and observe the yellow soap bubbles dissolving... ... You are innocent... ... You are innocent... ...

... ... Your deep inner self memorizes everything... ... Deep inside, you know that you can actually exhale all disturbing thoughts and feelings, today and every day in your life... ... You also know that everything you let go of is replaced by new, helpful, constructive thoughts... ... Today you can feel it... ... So you can also feel it any other day in your life... ... Whenever you want, you simply close your eyes briefly and

exhale everything disturbing as colored soap bubbles... ...
Just like today, they burst and dissolve... ... just like today...
... And you feel new strength... ...

#6

You want to let go of the past today... ... Everything from the past is a part of you and will accompany you throughout your life... ... in your memory... ... That's okay... ... But it wasn't the memory that burdened you, it was the feelings associated with it... ... maybe disappointment... ... or anger... ... maybe bitterness... ... or the desire for reparation... ... the deep wish to relive everything and do it differently... ...

... ... You have thought about so many things and imagined... ... always thinking: What if? ... ... But that was exactly the holding on that made your life so difficult... ... You can learn from memories... ... and you have already learned everything there was to learn... ... Now you can leave the memory and simultaneously let go... ... Now is the time to say goodbye to the what-if and focus on what is truly important... ... looking forward... ... shaping your life here and now, and every day... ...

Deep inside you, there is a place of clarity... ... At this place, there is only white, pure light... ... You stand at this place and see only light all around you... ... Let this image become very clear... ... white light around you... ... only light everywhere... ... Immerse yourself completely in the image of pure white light and perfect inner freedom... ...

... ... The more intensely you imagine the white light, the easier it is to create the feeling of inner freedom in this very moment... ... Now, in relaxation and calm, it is quite easy to feel the sense of inner freedom... ... because now everything feels calm... ... all problems are far away, because now it's only about your calmness... ... Now is time just for you... ... time just for you... ... Everywhere around you is white, pure light... ... Let it become clearer in your imagination... ... before your inner eye... ... white light and calm... ... white light and relaxation... ... white light and freedom... ... freedom... ...

... ... The ground under your feet seems to be made of glass... ... you can see through it... ... infinitely deep... ... But even there, you see only pleasant, white light... ... down to the infinite depth, white light... ... You look up and see only light above you as well... ... It is everywhere... ... bright and clear and very pleasant... ... It envelops you and gives you clarity and openness...

... ... You see a glass wall in front of you... ... You can look through it and see only light behind the wall... ... It is beautiful at the place of clarity... ... so pure... ... so free... ... so bright and clear... ... so distinct... ... You look at the wall in front of you once more... ... Slowly, writing appears on it in thick, clear outlines that become more distinct... ... You can recognize the writing... ... You can read it clearly... ... On the glass wall in front of you, at the place of clarity, it says... ... The past is over - The future belongs to you... ...

Let these words simply flow into you... ... Let them take effect and give yourself calm and mindfulness... calm and mindfulness... ... ... The past is over - The future belongs to you... ... Embrace yourself internally and feel the effect of the words you can read on the glass wall in front of you... ... The past is over - The future belongs to you... ...

... ... Everywhere is only white, clear, and pure light... ... and these words... ... The past is over - The future belongs to you... ...

This place of clarity is deep within you and the writing is there every day... ... Deep inside you, you read it every day... ... This way, you remind yourself every day that you can always let go... ... again and again... ... and it is really simple... ... a glance in the mirror is enough... ... Every morning when you look in the mirror, it is as if you are standing in front of the glass wall at the place of clarity and reading these words... ... The past is over - The future belongs to you... ... Every glance in the mirror reminds you... ... The past is over - The future belongs to you... ...

#7

Ideomotoric refers to the phenomenon where our body follows our feelings and thoughts with movements. In everyday life, this following manifests as body posture, muscle tension, and movement patterns of a person, which naturally change with the mood and thoughts. In trance, ideomotoric signals can be used to obtain information that the client cannot actively communicate. The subconscious can, for example, answer questions with an agreed finger signal. Naturally, ideomotoric reactions can also be used suggestively, for example in arm levitations and catalepsy. Such an approach, which I also apply in the following text, strengthens confidence in hypnosis and in one's ability to change, thereby promoting therapy.

You have often dealt with the past... ... have understood how things happened in your past and why everything happened the way it did... ... Many things have become clear to you... ... but some things may still be unclear or even puzzling... ...

... ... You have also realized... ... that we cannot understand everything and cannot analyze everything... ... Sometimes our task is to accept... ... because you can't change the past anyway... ... So you focus on more important things... ... on accepting and learning... ... You try to accept what happened as part of your journey... ... and you repeatedly set yourself to learn from the events and happenings... ... so that you can take even better care of yourself... ... so that you can draw your lessons and conclusions from the events of your life... ...

... ... In all these important learning processes, what your memory has stored helps you... ... that's enough, you don't need more... ... Now it can help you if you let go of the past... ... You can view and reconsider it at any time... ... It will be much easier if you first really let it go, so that you become free... ... free from bitterness or anger... ... free from thoughts of revenge or retribution... ... free for new paths and free for your own ideas... ...

... ... You have often wished the past was far away... ... so that you can feel free... ... Then the memory always came back, but it was not the memory that burdened you... ... It was the unresolved feelings... ... It was the longing to somehow change everything... ... the desire for reparation... ... or the help of fate to undo everything... ... Sometimes you felt like all the past was constantly with you... ... as if you just couldn't let it go... ... But today you do just that... ... You finally let go because today you are ready for it... ... You let go and your inner self helps you with it... ... You let go and can even feel the letting go... ... Your inner self shows you that you can let go... ... Your body shows you that you are letting go... ... Your hands will show you in a few moments... ...

... ... Then your hands will be free again and you can take hold of something new... ... can take something new into your hands... ... can walk your path... ... because your hands are free again... ... because your inner self is free and open again... ... because you have let go... ... have let go of the past... ... Today is the day you can accomplish this... ... exactly today is the right day for it... ...

... ... Now place your arms loosely beside your body... ... Make sure you are very comfortable... ... Just like that... ... and close your hands into a loose fist... ...

... ... Then think once more about the past that burdened you so much... ... Imagine it again, let your memory come up again, especially if it was painful... ... and the more intensely you think about it, the tighter your hands close... ... The longer you think about the past, the tighter your hands close into clenched fists... ... your hands close tighter and tighter... ... tighter and tighter... ...

... ... [Observe the client's hands, which close more tightly. Be careful to only suggest closing the hands until the fists are tightly closed. Please do not overdo it!] ... ...

... ... And now imagine that all the past that has stored itself in your inner self and disturbs you is loosening and flowing freely through your body... ... Maybe you know that not only our hands or our thoughts can hold on, but our entire body... ... memories, feelings, and thoughts are stored all over our body... ... we want to release the disturbing ones today... ... in this very moment... ... With the power of your thoughts, you can set your inner self to release all disturbing things and let them flow through your body... ... Maybe you can even feel it, like a breath of air or like a warm flow through your body... ... maybe cool... ... or you feel a tingling that shows you that disturbing thoughts and feelings are indeed loosening now... ... Maybe you can feel it... ... or you feel it a bit later, in a few moments... ... Then all that has loosened flows over your shoulders into your arms... ... to your hands... ... Your hands now let go of the past... ... In the process, your hands open slowly, at exactly the pace your inner self needs to let go of the past now... ... Your hands open and you let go of the past... ...

... ... [Observe the client's hands, which slowly open. Please give the client some time to internally set to let go. Help with simple suggestions if the hands do not open.] ... ...

... ... Your hands open more and more and even stretch out so that all disturbing things from the past can actually flow away... ...

... ... Your inner self firmly imprints that you are now free and can walk new paths... ... and whenever you want to strengthen the feeling of inner freedom, you can simply close your hands into fists and open them slowly and consciously... ... In the process, you breathe out deeply and then feel the inner liberation... ... You can do this any day of your life if you want... ... whenever you want... ... and wherever you want... ... It's very simple...

#8

You are here today to deal with your memories, especially the events that have burdened you and held you back repeatedly... ... Everything that lies in our memory can be found in our body... ... also what is deep in our soul can be found in our body... ... Every thought, every mood... ... every single feeling manifests in our body... ... shows up there as pressure... ... as tension... ... as a strange feeling... ... sometimes even as pain... ... or just as a strange tingling... ... So if you can clearly feel your body, you can also achieve everything you have set out to do... ... understand everything... ... and change everything... ... let go of everything you want to hand over to the past to be free and open again... ...

... ... Somewhere in your body is also the tormenting memory that has made you dwell on events of the past over and over again... ... There is also this pattern that has led you to hold on to old experiences over and over again... ... Let's call it your past pattern... ... It sits deep inside you and works from there without you noticing... ... But by now you know it... ... You have long understood that this special pattern must exist... ... You have accepted that it is there... ... At the same time, you have set out to find it and dissolve it... ...

... ... It is anchored in your feelings and thoughts, but also in your body... ... You can feel it in your body... ... Maybe you know that you can physically feel everything that belongs to you when you come to rest, like now... ... and focus on your body... ... like now... ... Of course, you have experienced in your everyday life how your past pattern can affect you, but it also shows up in your body... ... just differently... ... as tension... ... as warmth or cold... ... as pressure or in some other way... ... All patterns that we carry deep within us show up most clearly at a specific spot in our body... ... as a signal that we can perceive... ... So in your body, there is also a signal of your past pattern that can warn you... ... so that you don't fall into the trap of brooding or struggling... ... so that you can take better care of yourself... ... You just need to recognize this spot, then you can work on it and build a new pattern... ...

... ... Now direct your attention to your body and feel your body... ... Scan down from your head to your feet, as if you were standing next to yourself and could look at your body... ... and find this special spot... ... Find this spot that feels different because your past pattern is there... ...

... ... In your imagination, stand next to yourself and look at your body to find this special spot now... ... It is marked with a thick red dot... ... You see it before your inner eye... ... Just look at your body... ... Wherever this dot may be, it is exactly the spot on your body where your past pattern has settled... ...

You find it... ... It is marked in red and it feels different... ... maybe just a bit colder or warmer... ... maybe as a tingling... ... or as a slight goosebump that suddenly forms... ... Wherever this spot is... ... There your past pattern shows itself through a physical signal... ... right there... ... But even if you haven't found it... ... It is there... ... Then just take the spot that comes to your mind spontaneously... ... wherever that is... ...

... ... Feel deeper and deeper into it... ... Go all the way into this feeling... ... whatever it may be... ... It is your past pattern that you feel there... ... Go deeper and deeper into this spot on your body and feel the signals from your body more and more clearly... ... Maybe it feels strenuous or burdensome... ... Maybe you thought you had already overcome it more... ... Don't worry, because here you mainly feel the pattern that led to your holding on to the past and thus often to stagnation... ...

... ... Now focus all your attention and all your mindfulness and loving care on exactly this spot on your body and connect with the inner pattern that lies there... ... Imagine a small fresh spring beginning to bubble up from this spot... ... cool fresh water bubbles from this spring and simply dissolves the old pattern... ... The water from the beautiful spring cleanses your body... ... dissolves the old pattern and lets it simply flow away... ...

You are standing next to yourself and can observe it... ... All the old patterns of holding on just flow away... ... like sand being washed away by the flowing spring water until the water is clear and pure again... ... This clarity can encompass your entire body because you bring this mindfulness... ... this turning towards yourself... ... More and more old entanglements dissolve and are replaced by new patterns of self-care and mindfulness... ... Everywhere where the past pattern was recently, you find more and more love from you for yourself... ... more and more love from you for yourself... ... your self-love and mindfulness... ... your self-love and mindfulness... ... Continue to breathe calmly and evenly and trust in the power within you... ... Everywhere where the past pattern was recently, you find more and more love from you for yourself... ... more and more love from you for yourself... ... your self-love and mindfulness... ... your self-love and mindfulness... ...

... ... You feel the change in your body and make it clear to yourself that your body can always show you how you are feeling... ... especially the feelings that you couldn't always feel so well in everyday life... ... Now you can, because you know that your body helps you... ... So every day you pay attention to your body and ask yourself already in the morning when you get up how your body feels today... ... It shows you when you need to take better care of yourself...

#9

You go into the land of dreams... ... You are standing in a meadow and looking around... ... You see this mirror that stands in the middle of the meadow... ... You walk towards the mirror and look into it... ... You see your reflection... ... You might see many things that you don't like... ... maybe you even have criticism or a bad opinion of yourself... ... Maybe there are also great things that you notice... ... maybe you like yourself for one thing or another... ... and maybe many things are just mixed up... ... and you don't really know yet if you should like the person in the mirror or if you even have an opinion about the person in the mirror who is you... ...

Then you look to your left... ... standing on your left side is a child... ... maybe five or six years old... ... or a bit younger or older... ... And you ask the child at your side: "Who are you?" ... ... It looks at you in amazement and says: "Don't you know? ... ... Don't you remember me? ... ... Have you really forgotten me? ... ... You say: "I think I have... ... because I don't know you" ... ... The child looks at you with big eyes and says: "But I am you! ... ... I am the child within you... ... your inner child" ... ... And then you remember... ...

... ... You recognize that it looks just like you did... ... back when you were much smaller... ... But the child is sad and tells you about all the bad and sad things it experienced in its life... ... You hear your own story... ... Your inner child tells you about you...

And because it looks so sad, you take the child in your arms... ... You comfort the small child... ... which is also yourself... ... With all your good qualities... ... with all your strength and care, which you often have for others who are doing poorly, you comfort the small child... ... You hug and stroke it... ... You hold it very, very tightly in your arms...

And you know that you are good at this for other people... ... that you can comfort others and help them... ... and here you do it with yourself... ... with the part of you that now needs your help... ... that you can now love...

And you say: "I will never leave you alone again. Believe me, I will take care of you. Because who could be closer to me than you? Who could need me more than you, my child?" ...

You take your inner child by both hands and you begin to dance and sing... ... hand in hand, like happy friends... ... You play together and toss a colorful ball back and forth... ... The ball is painted with the bright colors of the rainbow... ... and you toss it to each other... ... It is feather-light... ... just as light as you are... ...

In this colorful ball is everything you have together... ... your past... ... everything you both have experienced... ... and you handle it lightly and carefree... ... playfully... ... In doing so, you feel very closely connected... ... You as the adult and you as the small child within you... ... Then you feel how wonderful it is to meet yourself here... ... and how glad you are that the child has found you now... ... It is very easy for you to comfort it for all that has happened in your past because for the child it is the present... ... You comfort the child as if it were another person... ... Because you are good at that... ... being there for others... ... And here you can do it for this small and sad child... ... You have made it happy again... ... simply by loving it...

And yet it is different than usual... ... because that is yourself... ... as a child within you... ... It is yourself you are comforting... ... You are the one playing and tossing the colorful ball with the rainbow colors back and forth... ... It is yourself who is now light and carefree, unburdened and free dealing with yourself... ... It is yourself who is loving you right now...

And then you look up at the sky... ... The view hasn't been this clear and the weather this beautiful for a long time... ... a wonderful day for you... ... And you think about how it would be if it were always like this... ... if you could be happy and cheerful with yourself... ... with the child within you and with everything you are... ... any time you feel like it... ... You consider whether you will succeed again or if you will soon forget the child again...

Then you remember that you have always been able to take good care of others... ... your whole life long... ... Even if you were sometimes selfish or neglected someone...

Then you still worried about them... ... had a bad conscience...

And you consider whether you can muster your strength for yourself... ... every day a little...

And you turn to the child who is still at your side and looking at you laughing... ... You say: "I want to always take care of you... ... I want to always love you... ... because you are me and I am you... ... And we are always together... ... even if I haven't seen you so often... ... and almost forgot your face...

The child, which is yourself, looks at you laughing, and asks you: "But what if I am naughty... ... if I do something... ... if I do something that brings you trouble... ... will you still love me then?" ...

And you as the adult answer the child: "But of course, my child... ... especially then... ... because then you need me even more...

And then you promise each other that you will always love each other and that you will never forget each other... ... You hug each other tightly and hold each other lovingly...

... ... Then you think that you can meet your inner child every day and help it again and again... ... Fantasy and reality are much closer together than you thought... ... You think about the fact that the land of dreams is deep within you. It has always been there. I'm just telling you about it...

#10

You go into the land of dreams and see many large crystal balls in front of you... so large that you can even go inside them... like into a large room of a house... And all these balls are lined up next to each other... Each ball represents a year of your life... And you can visit all the balls... or as many as you want... And today it is about a specific ball... maybe you already know which one it is... Or you don't know exactly what you can't let go of... Maybe you have a feeling that there are unresolved things... without knowing exactly what they are... or where you can find them... Or you know exactly in which time there is still something to be done... And yet you are not sure if this holding on does not come from an even earlier time... that may lie much further back... You stand before these balls that are lined up next to each other... at the far right end of this row of balls you stand... And then you go into the far right ball... the ball of the present... In this ball, there is a mirror... You look into it and you see yourself... And to the right and left of the mirror stand the people and the situations that play a role in your life today... You meet them every day or they are within reach... You can clarify with them every day what is still to be discussed... But today you go further... So you go into the next ball and stand before the mirror again and look at yourself... And you go further into the next ball... and from ball to ball... you will gradually get younger... because each ball stands for a year of your life... You can stay in each ball for a short while and look at yourself... in the mirror... and you see yourself getting younger...

Maybe you will also get smaller, because your journey goes back to your childhood... Quite on its own, you feel when you have arrived in the right time... in the time where you still want to let go of something... something that still occupies you... or bothers you... or something that still makes you suffer... How old are you? ... How are you? ... Which situation or event has brought you here? ... What feeling is it that connects you to this time? ... You see yourself in the mirror... and to the right and left of this mirror, you see the situations and people that belong to this time... Some people may still be close to you or closely connected to you today... Others may not play a big role in your life anymore... Others may not be alive anymore...

They have made this time journey with you and are now standing there as they did then... at that time you are thinking about now... where you now stand... in this crystal ball... Then you think again about how it was... what you experienced and what you felt... You see again how the others who are there now behaved... under whom you may have suffered... who stood by you... And you remember what it did to you...

And gradually a feeling arises for what keeps you stuck in this time... You remember the unresolved... or also what you couldn't resolve... Because you were perhaps too small... or too weak to help yourself... or others... And you couldn't be helped either... at least not in the way you needed... The comfort you needed and sought could not be given to you... And if there was someone who could have given it to you... someone who could have looked out for you or comforted you... then this person didn't do it any better than how they did... even if that may have hurt you a lot... If there is this person, you can talk to them now... You can tell them that you suffered and that you needed more... And maybe this person can now give you the comfort you didn't get back then... simply in your imagination...

... Maybe your tormentors are there too... those under whom you suffered... You hand them over with all their faults and shortcomings... with all their bad deeds to this past... You can say something to them if you want...

You make it clear to yourself once more that you are here today to make your inner peace... Peace with your past... to let go... You see that what you couldn't get back then, you can't pick up afterward... but you can still feel relief... Because now you see that it couldn't have been any different back then... even if they were terrible things that happened to you... or were done to you... Even if what happened may not be excusable... it is still true that it didn't happen any other way back then... whoever made mistakes at that time... Maybe these people have learned from it... to not do it that way again... But now you say goodbye to this time... to the situations and experiences... to the people... whether they were tormentors or your helpers... All stay in that time... You have learned from this time and made much good out of it... even if you don't always feel that way... Your suffering originated back then... and your holding on that disturbs and burdens you so much... But you also developed many of your good qualities back then... maybe the ability to take care of others... to listen to others... to comfort them... to be a helper yourself... or whatever else belongs to your good qualities... You would have liked to develop these in a gentle way... without your own suffering... But your story was different... You say goodbye now, because you know you can keep all your good qualities... even or especially by letting go of the past now... The feelings that belong to that time, you leave there in the ball... because that's where they belong... It is enough if you bring them along as a memory... You go back through the balls and get bigger and older... You return from ball to ball back to your present... You are back in the ball of today and return...

...... Then you think that maybe it's not just like this in the land of dreams, but also in your everyday life... ... Fantasy and reality are much closer together than you thought... ... You think about the fact that the land of dreams is deep within you. It has always been there. I'm just telling you about it...

Overview of All Titles in the Series "Ten Hypnoses"

Volume 1: Smoking Cessation
Volume 2: Anxiety and Restlessness
Volume 3: Burnout
Volume 4: Reducing Overweight
Volume 5: Coping with the Past
Volume 6: Suicidal Thoughts and Attempts
Volume 7: Psycho-Oncology
Volume 8: Obsessions and Tics
Volume 9: Self-Confidence and Decision-Making
Volume 10: Grief Work
Volume 11: Psychosomatics
Volume 12: Chronic Pain
Volume 13: Depressive Thoughts
Volume 14: Panic Attacks
Volume 15: Domestic Violence, Victim Support
Volume 16: Post-Traumatic Stress
Volume 17: Exam Anxiety and Stage Fright
Volume 18: Anti-Violence Training, Offender Support
Volume 19: Addiction Tendencies
Volume 20: Social Phobia and Fear of Contact
Volume 21: Nail Biting
Volume 22: Self-Awareness and Self-Love
Volume 23: Teeth Grinding and Night Clenching
Volume 24: Feelings of Guilt
Volume 25: Fear in Crowds
Volume 26: Fear of Flying, Aviophobia
Volume 27: Fear in Enclosed Spaces, Claustrophobia
Volume 28: Tinnitus, Ear Noises
Volume 29: Fear of Heights
Volume 30: Neurodermatitis

Volume 31: Finding Inner Balance
Volume 32: Overcoming Loneliness
Volume 33: Fear of Illness, Hypochondria
Volume 34: Anticipatory Anxiety, Fear of Fear
Volume 35: Jealousy in Relationships
Volume 36: Driving Anxiety
Volume 37: New Start after Separation
Volume 38: Fear of Injections
Volume 39: Heart Anxiety Neurosis
Volume 40: Overcoming Resentment and Anger
Volume 41: Resolving Blockages and Positive Thinking
Volume 42: Stress Reduction, Stress Management
Volume 43: Body Relaxation
Volume 44: Deep Relaxation
Volume 45: Fear of the Dark
Volume 46: Falling Asleep and Staying Asleep
Volume 47: Compulsive Buying
Volume 48: Restless Legs Syndrome
Volume 49: Bulimia
Volume 50: Anorexia
Volume 51: Overcoming Nightmares
Volume 52: Imagined Deformity
Volume 53: Overcoming Distrust, Finding Trust
Volume 54: Processing Failures
Volume 55: Humiliation, Emotional Hurt
Volume 56: Distressing Compassion, Vicarious Suffering
Volume 57: Self-Forgiveness
Volume 58: Self-Awareness, Self-Confidence
Volume 59: Saying No
Volume 60: Assertiveness
Volume 61: Setting Boundaries and Self-Assertion
Volume 62: Decision-Making Ability

Volume 63: Success Orientation
Volume 64: Ruminating, Circular Thinking
Volume 65: Accepting Pregnancy
Volume 66: Birth Preparation
Volume 67: Spiritual Opening
Volume 68: Joy of Life and Inner Lightness
Volume 69: Patience and Inner Peace
Volume 70: Fibromyalgia and Rheumatism
Volume 71: Irritable Bowel Syndrome, Crohn's Disease
Volume 72: Fear of Nausea, Emetophobia
Volume 73: Stuttering and Cluttering, Speech Flow Disorders
Volume 74: Concentration and Knowledge Anchoring
Volume 75: Vitality and Spontaneity
Volume 76: Searching for Meaning and Finding Goals
Volume 77: Life Crises, Life Events
Volume 78: Workaholism, Goal Obsession
Volume 79: Helper Syndrome, Helpless Helpers
Volume 80: Medication Abuse
Volume 81: Gambling Addiction
Volume 82: Internet Addiction, Smartphone Addiction
Volume 83: Hoarding Disorder, Compulsive Collecting
Volume 84: Conspiracy Thoughts, Overvalued Ideas
Volume 85: Fear of Operations and Treatments
Volume 86: Fear of Aging
Volume 87: Travel Anxiety
Volume 88: Anxiety When Urinating, Paruresis
Volume 89: Fear of Intimacy and Togetherness
Volume 90: Fear of Blushing
Volume 91: Coming Out in Homosexuality
Volume 92: Charisma Training
Volume 93: Migraines and Chronic Headaches
Volume 94: Overcoming Allergies, Bronchial Asthma

Volume 95: Normalizing Blood Pressure
Volume 96: Compulsive Perfectionism
Volume 97: Sports Hypnosis, Motivation
Volume 98: Sports Hypnosis, Performance Enhancement
Volume 99: Determination and Focus
Volume 100: Encountering the Inner Child
Volume 101: Cravings, Binge Eating
Volume 102: Stimulating Metabolism
Volume 103: Bipolar Mood Swings
Volume 104: Borderline, Identity Crises
Volume 105: Hypomania, Euphoria, Mania
Volume 106: Restlessness, Agitation
Volume 107: Nervous Breakdown
Volume 108: Adjustment Disorders
Volume 109: Self-Alienation, Depersonalization
Volume 110: Ending Self-Pity
Volume 111: Primary Gain of Illness
Volume 112: Secondary Gain of Illness
Volume 113: Bullying, Victim Support
Volume 114: Letting Go of Envy and Jealousy
Volume 115: Fear of Spiders, Arachnophobia
Volume 116: Fear of Dogs or Cats
Volume 117: Fear of Strangers, Xenophobia
Volume 118: Excessive Worries, Generalized Anxiety
Volume 119: Strengthening Sense of Responsibility
Volume 120: Unrequited Love, Heartache
Volume 121: Work-Life Balance
Volume 122: Letting Go of Unattainable Goals
Volume 123: Allowing and Accepting Help
Volume 124: Letting Go of Adult Children
Volume 125: Tourette Syndrome
Volume 126: Life Changes and New Starts

Volume 127: Accepting Life in a Wheelchair
Volume 128: Understanding and Overcoming Homesickness
Volume 129: Understanding and Overcoming Wanderlust
Volume 130: Dizziness, Meniere's Disease
Volume 131: Overcoming Aggression
Volume 132: Cutting and Self-Harm
Volume 133: Hair Pulling, Trichotillomania
Volume 134: Postpartum Depression
Volume 135: For Relatives of Dementia Patients
Volume 136: Self-Harm, Artificial Disorders
Volume 137: Activating Self-Healing Powers
Volume 138: Preventing Depression Relapse
Volume 139: Reactive Psychoses, Follow-Up
Volume 140: Obsessive Thoughts and Impulses
Volume 141: Compulsive Checking
Volume 142: Compulsive Counting, Symmetry Obsession
Volume 143: Compulsive Washing, Cleanliness Obsession
Volume 144: Compulsive Questioning
Volume 145: Dissociative Paralysis
Volume 146: Phantom Pain
Volume 147: Overcoming Complaining
Volume 148: Hay Fever, Pollen Allergy
Volume 149: Sexual Abuse, Victim Support
Volume 150: Standing Strong Against Sexism, #metoo
Volume 151: Binge Eating
Volume 152: Overcoming Thoughts of Revenge
Volume 153: Detachment from the Aggressor, Stockholm Syndrome
Volume 154: Courage to Separate
Volume 155: Chronic Fatigue, Exhaustion
Volume 156: Fear of the Future, Existential Anxiety
Volume 157: Excessive Worry About Children
Volume 158: Fear of Failure

Volume 159: Ending Distrust and Control
Volume 160: Dejection, Dysphoria
Volume 161: Boreout, Chronic Boredom
Volume 162: Bipolar Disorders, Relapse Prevention
Volume 163: Mania, Relapse Prevention
Volume 164: Nihilism, Feelings of Worthlessness
Volume 165: Thumb Sucking
Volume 166: Being Brave
Volume 167: Being Proud
Volume 168: Overcoming Shyness
Volume 169: Being Able to Delegate Responsibility
Volume 170: Being Able to Show Emotions
Volume 171: Letting Go of Guilt, Victim Support
Volume 172: Processing Guilt, Offender Support
Volume 173: Mood Swings, Cyclothymia
Volume 174: Lack of Drive, Vital Sadness
Volume 175: Hearing Voices with Reality Reference
Volume 176: Confident Communication
Volume 177: Standing Up for Oneself
Volume 178: Taking New Paths
Volume 179: Confident Job Application
Volume 180: No Longer Being Taken Advantage Of
Volume 181: End of Submissiveness
Volume 182: Depressive Numbness
Volume 183: Mood Drops, Affective Incontinence
Volume 184: Mood Instability
Volume 185: Somatoform Disorders
Volume 186: Stomach Ulcer, Psychosomatic
Volume 187: Accepting Amputation
Volume 188: Overcoming and Letting Go of Hatred
Volume 189: Ending Accusations
Volume 190: Allowing Tears, Being Able to Cry

Volume 191: Finding and Sorting Repressed Feelings
Volume 192: Somatoform Pain
Volume 193: Living Autonomously
Volume 194: Anhedonia, Joylessness
Volume 195: Persistent Sadness
Volume 196: Obesity, Food Addiction
Volume 197: Parents of Abused Children
Volume 198: Letting Go and Letting Be
Volume 199: Childhood Sexual Abuse
Volume 200: Fear of Loss

www.ingramcontent.com/pod-product-compliance
Lightning Source LLC
Chambersburg PA
CBHW030501220526
45464CB00006B/2608